The Vibrant Recipe Co

Healthy and Tasty Keto Recipes to Avoid Carbohydrates and Manage Your Weight

Sebastian Booth

Table of contents

Baked Chicken Thighs With Lemon Butter Caper Sauce

Marcos: Fat 71% | Protein 26% | Carbs 3%

Prep time: 15 minutes | Cook time: 30 minutes | Serves 4

Sometimes, we are hungry for a tasty meal, but never have the time for it, or do we? That's right my dear hungry friend. These delicious chicken thighs alongside with lemon butter caper sauce could be prepared in less than an hour. So get your ingredients ready and prepare yourself for an exquisite meal packed with flavor.

1 teaspoon sea salt

½ teaspoon ground black pepper

1 tablespoon Italian seasoning

1 tablespoon garlic powder

2 pounds (907 g) bone-in chicken thighs, skin-on

2 tablespoons olive oil

3 tablespoons butter

2 tablespoons lemon juice

1 lemon, divided into wheels

SERVING:

2 ounces (57 g) leafy vegetables

1. Preheat the oven to 400°F (205°C).

2. Use salt, pepper, Italian seasoning and garlic powder to season the thighs on both sides.

3. Heat the olive oil in a large skillet over medium heat. Add the chicken thighs, skin side down, and cook for about 5 minutes until the skin turns crispy and nice.

4. Flip the chicken thighs over and put the skillet into the preheated oven. Bake for 15 to 20 minutes until the chicken is cooked through.

5. Remove the chicken from the oven to a plate and set aside.

6. Add the butter and lemon juice to the same skillet over medium-high for 2 to 3 minutes, and keep stirring until the sauce gets thickened. Scarp any leftover bits stuck to the bottom of the skillet with a spatula.

7. Pour the sauce over the chicken and garnish with lemon wheels, then serve with leafy vegetables.

STORAGE: Store in a sealed airtight container in the fridge for up to 5 days or in your freezer for about 1 month.

REHEAT: Microwave, covered, until the desired temperature is reached or reheat in a frying pan or instant pot, covered, on medium.

SERVE IT WITH: It could be served with the vegan kale salad.

PER SERVING

calories: 635 | fat: 50.3g | total carbs: 5.5g | fiber: 0.8g | protein:38.6g

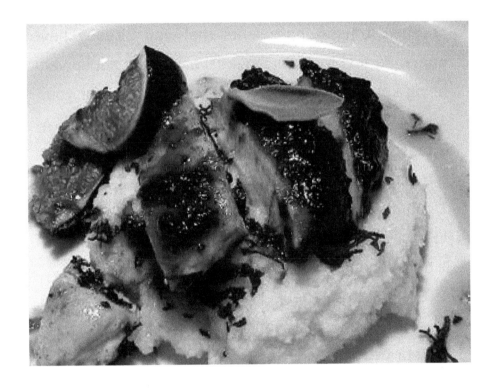

Grilled Spiced Chicken

Macros: Fat: 78% | Protein: 21% | Carbs: 1%

Prep time: 15 minutes | Cook time: 20 minutes | Serves 10

A grill and a generous heart are all you need to make this dish a reality, don't forget the ingredients too! This grilled spiced chicken dish is a quick and easy dish to cook because it uses ingredients that you already have at home. Perfect for busy weekdays with the added value of being keto-friendly, this dish is the best bet for you.

1 teaspoon garlic powder

1 teaspoon ground paprika

1 teaspoon poultry seasoning

1 cup of olive oil

½ cup apple cider vinegar

1 tablespoon salt

1 teaspoon black pepper

10 skinless chicken thighs

1. Pour the garlic powder, paprika, poultry seasoning, oil, vinegar, salt, and black pepper into a jar with a lid, cover the jar and shake it well to combine.

2. Put the chicken thighs on a baking dish and pour three-quarters of the powder mixture over them. Cover the dish with plastic wrap and put it in the

refrigerator to marinate for 8 hours, preferably overnight.

3. Preheat the grill to high heat.

4. Place the chicken on the grill to cook for 10 minutes on each side.

5. Transfer the chicken to a plate and brush with the remaining powder mixture, then serve.

STORAGE: Store in an airtight container in the fridge for up to 4 days or in the freezer for up to 1 month.

REHEAT: Microwave, covered, until the desired temperature is reached or reheat in a frying pan or air fryer / instant pot, covered, on medium.

SERVE IT WITH: To make this a complete meal, serve it with a bowl of green salad.

PER SERVING

calories: 615 | fat: 53.7g | total carbs: 1.2g | fiber: 0.2g | protein: 32.0g

Spicy Garlic Chicken Kebabs

Macros: Fat: 50% | Protein: 44% | Carbs: 6%

Prep time: 15 minutes | Cook time: 12 minutes | Serves 6

Chicken kebabs has always been a party pleaser but this spicy variation will kick your party up a notch. It can be stored and reheated which makes it a suitable leftover meal and can replace carb-laden snacks.

1 cup plain Greek yogurt

2 tablespoons freshly squeezed lemon juice, or more to taste

1 tablespoon kosher salt

1½ teaspoons ground cumin

1 teaspoon freshly ground black pepper

⅛ teaspoon ground cinnamon

2 tablespoons olive oil, divided

6 cloves garlic, minced

1 tablespoon red pepper flakes

1 teaspoon paprika

2½ pounds (1.1 kg) boneless, skinless chicken thighs, halved

SPECIAL EQUIPMENT:

4 long metal skewers

1. Mix the yogurt, lemon juice, kosher salt, cumin, black pepper, cinnamon, 1 tablespoon olive oil, garlic, red pepper flakes, and paprika together in a bowl.
2. Put the chicken in the marinade to coat, then cover the bowl with plastic wrap and refrigerate to marinate for 2 to 8 hours.
3. Preheat the grill to medium-high heat and brush the grill grates with the remaining olive oil.
4. Make the kebabs: Thread half of the chicken on two skewers and shape it into a thick log.
5. Put the kebabs on the grill and cook for 4 to 5 minutes. Flip the kebabs over and cook the for about 6 minutes more, or until cooked through and a meat thermometer inserted in the center registers 165ºF (74ºC).
6. Remove the kebabs from the grill and serve on a plate.

STORAGE: Store in an airtight container in the fridge for up to 4 days or in the freezer for up to 1 month.

REHEAT: Microwave, covered, until the desired temperature is reached or reheat in a frying pan or air fryer / instant pot, covered, on medium.

SERVE IT WITH: To make this a complete meal, serve it with a bowl of green salad.

PER SERVING

calories: 512 | fat: 28.5g | total carbs: 11.7g | fiber: 4.1g | protein: 56.3g

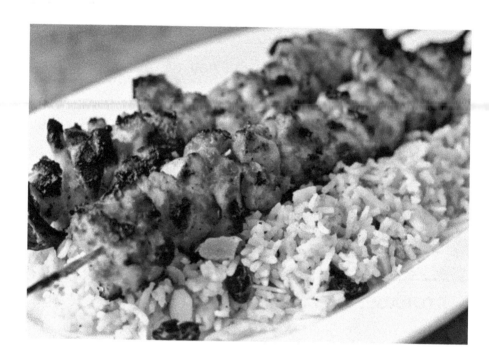

Cheesy Chicken Dish with Spinach

Macros: Fat: 54% | Protein: 40% | Carbs: 6%

Prep time: 10 minutes | Cook time: 15 minutes | Serves 4

This mouth-watering cheesy chicken dish with spinach and tomatoes is just bursting with flavorful deliciousness. It is a family favorite dish and can bring any boring dish to life. Dip your fork into this cheesy deliciousness and you certainly won't regret it.

2 tablespoons olive oil

1½ pounds (680 g) skinless, boneless chicken breast, thinly sliced

1 cup heavy cream

1 teaspoon garlic powder

1 teaspoon Italian seasoning

½ cup chicken broth

½ cup Parmesan cheese, grated

1 cup spinach, chopped

½ cup sun-dried tomatoes, chopped

1. Heat the olive oil in a large skillet over medium-high heat.
2. Add the chicken to the skillet and cook for 3 to 5 minutes on each side or until lightly browned. Transfer the chicken to a plate and set aside.

3. Pour the heavy cream in the skillet and add the garlic powder, Italian seasoning, chicken broth, and Parmesan cheese, then whisk well for 5 minutes or until the sauce starts to thicken.

4. Mix in the spinach and the tomatoes and cook on low heat for 1 minute. Put the chicken back into the skillet and cook for 2 to 3 minutes. Keep stirring during the cooking.

5. Remove from the heat and serve on plates.

STORAGE: Store in an airtight container in the fridge for up to 4 days or in the freezer for up to 1 month.

REHEAT: Microwave, covered, until the desired temperature is reached or reheat in a frying pan or instant pot, covered, on medium.

SERVE IT WITH: To make this a complete meal, serve it with Greek salad or coleslaw.

PER SERVING

calories: 437 | fat: 26.1g | total carbs: 7.7g | fiber: 1.2g | protein: 44.0g

Delicious Parmesan Chicken

Macros: Fat 75% | Protein 23% | Carbs 2%

Prep time: 20 minutes | Cook time: 8 minutes | Serves 4

The kids will enjoy this delicious Parmesan chicken especially for dinner. The chicken is enriched with essential nutrients from the cream, pork rinds, eggs, and Parmesan cheese. It is a fulfilling recipe for keto diet.

1 (8-ounce / 227-g) skinless, boneless chicken breast

1 tablespoon heavy whipping cream

1 egg

½ teaspoon salt

½ teaspoon red pepper flakes

1 ounce (28 g) grated Parmesan cheese

1½ ounces (43 g) crushed pork rinds

½ teaspoon ground black pepper

½ teaspoon garlic powder

½ teaspoon Italian seasoning

1 tablespoon butter

¼ cup shredded Mozzarella cheese

1. Start by preheating the oven's broiler and put the oven rack about 6 inches from the heat source.

2. On a flat work surface, slice the chicken breast horizontally through the middle, Pound the chicken to ½-inch thickness with a meat mallet.

3. In a bowl, beat the cream and the egg until smooth. Set aside.

4. In another bowl, combine the salt, red pepper flakes, Parmesan cheese, pork rinds, black pepper, garlic powder, and Italian seasoning. Transfer the breading mixture to a plate.

5. Dip the chicken into the egg mixture, then press the chicken into the breading mixture to coat thickly on both sides.

6. Melt the butter in a skillet over medium-high heat.

7. Cook the chicken for about 3 minutes per side, or until it is no longer pink and juices are clear.

8. Put the cooked chicken in a baking tray then top up with Mozzarella cheese.

9. Broil in the preheated oven for about 2 minutes until the cheese is barely brown and bubbly.

STORAGE: Store in an airtight container in the fridge for up to 1 week.

REHEAT: Microwave, covered, until the desired temperature is reached or reheat in a frying pan or air fryer, covered, on medium.

SERVE IT WITH: To make this a complete meal, serve the Parmesan chicken with zucchini noodles.

PER SERVING

calories: 492 | fat: 41.2g | total carbs: 2.5g | fiber: 0.4g | protein:28.1g

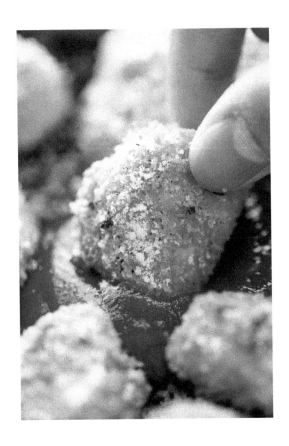

Michigander -Style Turkey
Macros: Fat 40% | Protein 59% | Carbs 1%

Prep time: 10 minutes | Cook time: 4 hours | Serves 16

Wondering what to prepare your entire family for dinner? Michigander-style turkey will sort out all your worries. During the last minutes of cooking, remember to remove the foil so that the turkey browns nicely.

1 (12-pound / 5.4-kg) whole turkey

6 tablespoons butter, divided

3 tablespoons chicken broth

4 cups warm water

2 tablespoons dried onion, minced

2 tablespoons dried parsley

2 tablespoons seasoning salt

1. Start by preheating the oven to 35 0°F (18 0°C).
2. Rinse the turkey and pat dry with paper towels.
3. Put the turkey on a roasting pan, then separate the skin over the breast to make pockets.
4. Put 3 tablespoons of butter into each pocket.
5. Mix the broth and water in a medium bowl.
6. Add the minced onion and parsley, then pour over the turkey. Sprinkle some salt on the turkey then cover with aluminum foil.

7. Bake in the preheated oven until the internal temperatures of the turkey reads 180°F (8 0℃), for about 4 hours.

8. When 45 minutes are remaining, remove the foil so that the turkey browns well.

9. Remove from the oven and serve warm.

STORAGE: Store in an airtight container in the fridge for up to 1 week

REHEAT: Microwave, covered, until the desired temperature is reached or reheat in an air fryer covered, on medium.

SERVE IT WITH: To make this a complete meal, serve the turkey with sautéed garlic kale and lemon.

PER SERVING

calories: 497 | fat: 22.1g | total carbs: 0.6g | fiber: 0g | protein: 73.8g

Keto Chicken Casserole

Macros: Fat 46% | Protein 46% | Carbs 8%

Prep time: 15 minutes | Cook time: 25 minutes | Serves 4

Keto chicken casserole is a recipe you have come across not once but several times. However, it is worth cooking over and over again because of its great taste and essential nutrients especially on keto diet. This recipe is perfect for dinner.

4 skinless, boneless chicken breast halves

¼ cup butter

1 tablespoon Italian seasoning

3 teaspoons minced garlic

½ cup grated Parmesan cheese

1 tablespoon lemon juice

½ cup heavy cream

1 (10 ¾ -ounce / 305-g) can condensed cream of mushroom soup

2 (13 ½ -ounce / 383-g) cans drained spinach

4 ounces (113 g) fresh sliced mushrooms

⅔ cup bacon bits

2 cups shredded Mozzarella cheese

1. Start by preheating the oven to 35 0 °F (18 0 °C), then put the chicken breast halves on a greased baking tray.
2. Bake in the preheated oven for 30 minutes until the juices are clear. Remove from the oven and put aside.
3. Increase the temperatures in the oven to 40 0 °F (20 5 °C).
4. Melt the butter in a medium saucepan over medium heat.
5. Add the Italian seasoning, garlic, Parmesan cheese, lemon juice, heavy cream, and mushroom soup, stirring continuously, for about 4 minutes. Set aside.
6. Place the spinach at the bottom of a baking dish.
7. Add the mushrooms then pour ½ of the mixture from the saucepan on top.
8. Place the chicken then pour the remaining sauce mixture.
9. Sprinkle the bacon bits then top with Mozzarella cheese.
10. Bake in the preheated oven for about 25 minutes until the chicken is lightly browned and the cheese is bubbly.
11. Remove form the oven and slice to serve.

STORAGE: Store in an airtight container in the fridge for up to 1 week

REHEAT: Microwave, covered, until the desired temperature is reached or reheat in an air fryer, covered, on medium.

SERVE IT WITH: To make this a complete meal, serve the chicken casserole with buttered mushrooms.

PER SERVING

calories: 717 | fat: 36.6g | total carbs: 21.3g | fiber: 6.3g | protein: 81.9g

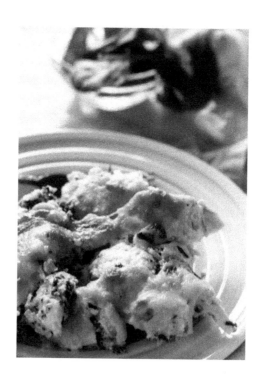

Almond Chicken Cordon Bleu

Macros: Fat 46% | Protein 52% | Carbs 2%

Prep time: 10 minutes | Cook time: 35 minutes | Serves 4

If you want to surprise your family with a unique and tasty chicken recipe, then go for almond chicken cordon bleu. The almond flavor gives the chicken a tasty approach that will leave you craving for more. For best results, use a chicken breast without bones.

2 tablespoons olive oil

4 skinless, boneless chicken breast halves

⅛ teaspoon ground black pepper

¼ teaspoon salt

6 slices Swiss cheese

4 slices cooked ham

½ cup almond meal

SPECIAL EQUIPMENT:

Toothpicks, soaked for at least 30 minutes

1. Start by preheating the oven to 35 0 °F (18 0 °C) then grease a baking sheet with olive oil.
2. On a flat work surface, using a meat mallet to pound the chicken until it is ¼-inch thickness.
3. Sprinkle the pepper and salt on each piece of the chicken evenly.

4. Put 1 slice of ham and 1 slice of cheese on each breast.

5. Roll each breast and tightly secure with a toothpick.

6. Arrange them on the prepared baking sheet and evenly sprinkle with the almond meal.

7. Bake in the preheated oven until cooked through, for about 35 minutes

8. Remove from the oven and top each breast with ½ cheese slice.

9. Return to the oven and bake for 5 minutes more, until the cheese is bubbly.

10. Remove from the oven and serve on plates.

STORAGE: Store in an airtight container in the fridge for up to 1 week

REHEAT: Microwave, covered, until the desired temperature is reached or reheat in an air fryer, covered, on medium.

SERVE IT WITH: To make this a complete meal, serve the almond chicken cordon bleu with saucy chili-garlic cucumber noodles

PER SERVING

calories: 532 | fat: 27.1g | total carbs: 3.4g | fiber: 0.4g | protein: 69.1g

Grilled Chicken Breast

Macros: Fat 34% | Protein 65% | Carbs 1%

Prep time: 15 minutes | Cook time: 20 minutes | Serves 4

If you are craving for some juicy grilled chicken while on keto diet then this grilled chicken breast is the best option. You can prepare this recipe for lunch or dinner and enjoy with your family.

1 tablespoon olive oil

1 teaspoon steak sauce

2 tablespoons keto-friendly mayonnaise

⅓ teaspoon liquid stevia

⅓ cup Dijon mustard

4 skinless, boneless chicken breast halves

1. Start by preheating the grill on medium heat and lightly grease the grill grate with olive oil.

2. Mix together the steak sauce, mayonnaise, stevia, and mustard in a bowl. Reserve some mustard sauce for basting in another bowl, then coat the chicken with the remaining sauce.

3. Grill the chicken for about 20 minutes until the juices are clear, flipping occasionally and basting frequently with the reserved sauce.

4. Remove from the grill and serve hot.

STORAGE: Store in an airtight container in the fridge for up to 1 week

REHEAT: Microwave, covered, until the desired temperature is reached or reheat in a frying pan or air fryer / instant pot, covered, on medium.

SERVE IT WITH: To make this a complete meal, serve the grilled chicken with creamy spinach dill.

PER SERVING

calories: 333 | fat: 12.6g | total carbs: 1.5g | fiber: 0.9g | protein: 54.3g

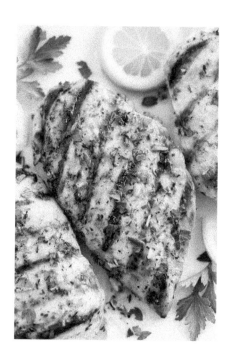

Bacon-Wrapped Chicken Breasts Stuffed with Spinach

Macros: Fat 59% | Protein 39% | Carbs 2%

Prep time: 25 minutes | Cook time: 1 hour | Serves 4

Trust me, this easy bacon-wrapped chicken breasts stuffed with spinach will become your family favorite! The flavor of the cheeses will bring you and your families tons of flavor. And the choice of spinach for this recipe will also increase the nutritional value of the meal.

1 (10-ounce / 284-g) package frozen chopped spinach, thawed and drained

½ cup mayonnaise, keto-friendly

½ cup feta cheese, shredded

2 cloves garlic, chopped

4 skinless, boneless chicken breasts

4 slices bacon

1. Preheat the oven to 375ºF (190ºC).

2. Combine the spinach, mayo, feta cheese, and garlic in a bowl, then set aside.

3. Cut the chicken crosswise to butterfly the chicken breasts, (butterfly cutting technique: not to cut the chicken breast through, leave a 1-inch space uncut

at the end of the chicken. So when flipping open the halved chicken breast, it resembles a butterfly.)

4. Unfold the chicken breasts like a book. Divide and arrange the spinach mixture over each breast, then wrap each breast with a slice of bacon and secure with a toothpick.

5. Arrange them in a baking dish, and cover a piece of aluminum foil. Place the dish in the preheated oven and bake for 1 hour or until the bacon is crispy and the juice of chicken breasts run clear.

6. Remove the baking dish from the oven and serve warm.

STORAGE: Store in an airtight container in the fridge for up to 4 days or in the freezer for up to 1 month.

REHEAT: Microwave, covered, until the desired temperature is reached or reheat in a frying pan or air fryer / instant pot, covered, on medium.

SERVE IT WITH: To make this a complete meal, serve them on a bed of greens or serve with a cherry tomato and zucchini salad.

PER SERVING

calories: 626 | fat: 41.3g | total carbs: 3.7g | fiber: 1.4g | protein: 61.2g

Rotisserie-Style Roast Chicken

Macros: Fat 64% | Protein 35% | Carbs 1%

Prep time:10minutes | Cook time: 5 hours | Serves 8

With minimal preparation and about 5 hours' cooking time,you can get that restaurant-style rotisserie chicken at home as you ever wish. It is super simple to make. No special skills are required. It is delicious and the leftovers are just as good the next day!

1 teaspoon onion powder

1 teaspoon white pepper

1 teaspoon dried thyme

½ teaspoon garlic powder

½ teaspoon cayenne pepper

1 teaspoons paprika

2 teaspoons salt

½ teaspoon black pepper

1 (4-pound / 1.8-kg) whole chickens, giblets removed, rinsed and pat dry

1 onion, quartered

1. Combine the onion powder, white pepper, thyme, garlic powder, cayenne pepper, paprika, salt, and black pepper in a bowl.

2. Rub the whole chicken with the powder mixture on all sides. Arrange the onion quarters into the cavity of the chicken.

3. Wrap the chicken with two layers of plastic and refrigerate for at least 4 hours.

4. Preheat the oven to 250ºF (120ºC).

5. Arrange the chicken in a baking pan and bake in the preheated oven for 5 hours or until a meat thermometer inserted in the center of the chicken reads at least 180ºF (82ºC).

6. Remove the chicken from the oven. Allow to cool for 10 minutes and slice to serve.

STORAGE: Store in an airtight container in the fridge for up to 4 days or in the freezer for up to 1 month.

REHEAT: Microwave, covered, until the desired temperature is reached or reheat in a frying pan or air fryer / instant pot, covered, on medium.

SERVE IT WITH: Easy lemon-ginger spinach is a perfect match for this dish, or you can have it with oven-roasted frozen broccoli cooked in the left juices. It will burst the flavors inside your mouth.

PER SERVING

calories: 484 | fat: 34.2g | total carbs: 2.2g | fiber: 0.6g | protein: 42.5g

Chicken Fajitas Bake

Macros: Fat 74% | Protein 21% | Carbs 5%

Prep time: 10 minutes | Cook time: 15 minutes |
Serves 4 to 6

This keto chicken casserole is the perfect low-carb meal
for the whole family. It has all of your favorite fajita
flavors all in one skillet. It is super simple, with only 7
main ingredients, and can be made in about 20 minutes.
This would be a great weeknight family-friendly keto
recipe. It's an easy keto recipe for beginners, too!

⅓ cup mayonnaise, keto-friendly

1 yellow onion, chopped

1 red bell pepper, chopped

1 rotisserie chicken breast, shred into bite-sized pieces

2 tablespoons Tex-Mex seasoning

2 tablespoons olive oil

5 ⅓ ounces (150 g) lettuce

7 ounces (198 g) cream cheese

Salt and freshly ground black pepper, to taste

7 ounces (198 g) shredded Cheddar cheese, divided

1. Preheat the oven to 400°F (205°C).

2. Add all the ingredients except for a third of the cheese
   to a lightly greased casserole dish. Stir to combine
   well.

3. Top the mixture with remaining cheese, then arrange the casserole dish in the preheated oven. Bake for 15 minutes or until lightly browned.
4. Remove the casserole dish from the oven and serve warm.

STORAGE: Store in an airtight container in the fridge for up to 4 days.

REHEAT: Microwave, covered, until the desired temperature is reached or reheat in a frying pan or air fryer / instant pot, covered, on medium.

SERVE IT WITH: To make this a complete meal, you can serve this casserole dish with leafy greens dressed in olive oil.

PER SERVING

calories: 526 | fat: 43.1g | total carbs: 7.0g | fiber: 1.5g | protein: 27.7g

Savoury And Sticky Baked Chicken Wings
Macros: Fat 37% | Protein 62% | Carbs 1%

Prep time: 5 minutes | Cook time: 45 minutes | Serves 4

These wings are great. There is a heat to them, but non-spice lovers enjoy them too because of the sweetness. They have a sweet, spicy, smoky flavor that will make you do a happy dance for sure! Made with a keto-friendly homemade marinade you can ensure there's no nasty preservatives or refined sugars in these bad boys!

2 pounds (907 g) chicken wings

1 teaspoon sea salt

SAUCE:

¾ cup coconut aminos

¼ teaspoon garlic powder

¼ teaspoon red pepper flakes

¼ teaspoon onion powder

¼ teaspoon ground ginger

1. Preheat oven to 450°F (235°C).
2. Arrange the chicken wings in a baking pan, skin side down. Make sure to keep a little distance between wings.

3. Sprinkle salt to season the wings, then bake in the preheated oven for 45 minutes or until crispy and cooked through.

4. Meanwhile, make the sauce: Warm a nonstick skillet over medium heat, then add the coconut aminos, garlic powder, red pepper flakes, onion powder, and ginger powder. Bring them to a simmer.

5. Reduce the heat to low and keep simmering. Stir the mixture constantly to combine well until the sauce is lightly thickened.

6. Arrange the chicken wings on a large serving dish. Pour the sauce over to coat the chicken wings and serve warm.

STORAGE: Store in an airtight container in the fridge for up to 4 days.

REHEAT: Microwave, covered, until the desired temperature is reached or reheat in a frying pan or air fryer / instant pot, covered, on medium.

SERVE IT WITH: Serve them with roasted Brussels sprout and rich cod fish soup.

PER SERVING

calories: 450 | fat: 18.5g | total carbs: 9.4g | fiber: 0.1g | protein: 69.2g

Low-Carb Chicken with Tricolore Roasted Veggies

Macros: Fat 71% | Protein 21% | Carbs 8%

Prep time: 15 minutes | Cook time: 30 minutes | Serves 8

It really is a beautiful and most colorful dish. So easy-to-make with lots of good flavor, and you can choose to cook it with either a whole chicken or chicken breasts.

TRICOLORE ROASTED VEGGIES:

8 ounces (227 g) mushrooms

1 pound (454 g) Brussels sprouts

8 ounces (227 g) cherry tomatoes

1 teaspoon dried rosemary

1 teaspoon sea salt

½ teaspoon ground black pepper

½ cup olive oil

FRIED CHICKEN:

4 chicken breasts

1 ounce (28 g) butter, for frying

Salt and freshly ground black pepper, to taste

4 ounces (113 g) herb butter, for serving

1. Preheat the oven to 400°F (205°C).

2. Arrange the mushrooms, Brussels sprouts, and cherry tomatoes in a baking pan.

3. Sprinkle with rosemary, salt, and ground black pepper. Pour the olive oil over. Stir to coat the veggies well.
4. Arrange the baking pan in the preheated oven and bake for about 20 minutes or until the Brussels spouts are wilted and the veggies are soft.
5. In the meantime, melt the butter in a nonstick skillet over medium heat, then place the chicken breasts in the pan. Sprinkle with salt and pepper.
6. Fry the chicken in the skillet for 8 to 10 minutes or until there is no pink on the chicken and the juices run clear.
7. Remove the baked veggies from the oven and serve with th e fried chicken.

STORAGE: Roasted vegetables can be stored in the refrigerator for 3 to 4 days. Store any leftover chicken in the fridge. This will store for up to three days.

REHEAT: Heat roasted vegetables again in a hot oven to keep them firm and crisp. A microwave will just turn them to mush. Spread the vegetables out on a baking sheet, drizzle them with olive oil, and bake at 450ºF (235ºC) for 4 or 5 minutes.

SERVE IT WITH: To make this a complete meal, you can serve it with with roasted Brussels sprout and rich sea white fish soup.

PER SERVING

calories: 390 | fat: 30.8g | total carbs: 10.4g | fiber: 3.1g | protein: 20.9g

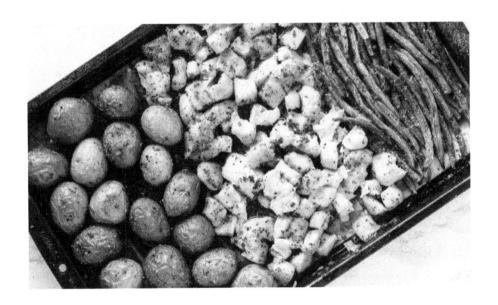

Cheese Stuffed Chicken Breast with Guacamole

Macros: Fat 69% | Protein 23% | Carbs 8%

Prep time: 20 minutes | Cook time: 20 minutes | Serves 6

This is a super delicious recipe. The taste of cheese with the flavor of the spiced chicken is balanced, and the cheese can be changed to Parmesan cheese for additional salty flavor. This is a meal with low budget to maintain a healthy body.

CHEESE STUFFED CHICKEN:

1 green bell pepper or red bell pepper, chopped

1 garlic clove, granulated

2 tablespoons olive oil

1½ pounds (680 g) chicken breasts

3 ounces (85 g) cream cheese

4 ounces (113 g) Cheddar cheese, shredded

2 tablespoons pickled jalapeños, finely chopped

½ teaspoon ground cumin

1 ginger, minced

Salt and freshly ground black pepper, to taste

SPECIAL EQUIPMENT:

4 toothpicks, soak in water for at least 30 minutes

FOR SERVING:

8 ounces (227 g) lettuce

1 cup sour cream

GUACAMOLE:

2 ripe avocados, peeled

½ lime, the juice

2 garlic cloves, minced

1 diced tomato

3 tablespoons olive oil

5 tablespoons fresh cilantro, finely chopped

Salt and freshly ground black pepper, to taste

1. Preheat the oven to 350°F (180°C).

2. Warm the olive oil in a nonstick skillet over medium heat. Add the garlic and bell pepper and sauté for about 3 minutes until the bell pepper is soft. Transfer to a bowl and allow to cool for 5 minutes.

3. Sprinkle the cheeses, jalapeños, cumin, and ginger in the bowl. Toss to combine well. Set aside.

4. Butterfly the chicken breasts by cutting them crosswise and leave a 1-inch space uncut at the end of the breasts.

5. Unfold the breasts on a clean working surface like a book, then divide and spread the cheese mixture in the breasts. Close the 'book' and secure each

chicken breast with a toothpick. Sprinkle with salt and pepper.

6. Arrange the stuffed chicken breasts in a lightly greased frying pan and fry for 8 minutes or until lightly browned. Place the fried chicken in a baking dish.

7. Pour the remaining cheese mixture over the chicken breasts and bake in the preheated oven for 20 minutes or until a meat thermometer inserted in the middle of the chicken reads at least 165ºF (74ºC).

8. Remove the tooth picks and serve with lettuce, guacamole, and sour cream.

GUACAMOLE:

1. Mash the guacamole with a fork in a large bowl. Top with lime juice and minced garlic.

2. Add tomato, olive oil and finely chopped cilantro. Season with salt and pepper, and blend well.

STORAGE: Chicken breast filled cheese with guacamole can be stored covered in the fridge for 2 up to 3 days, you can even freeze it in a freezer-safe container for up to 1 month.

REHEAT: Microwave, until it reaches the desired temperature.

SERVE IT WITH: To make it a complete meal, you can serve it with a mushroom and salmon salad and berry smoothie.

PER SERVING

calories: 599 | fat: 47.1g | total carbs: 13.5g | fiber: 5.9g | protein: 32.8g

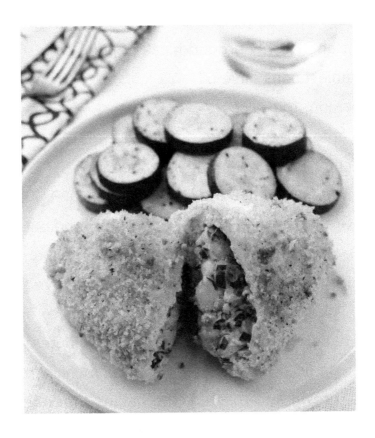

Garlic Chicken Low-Carb

Macros: Fat 66% | Protein 31% | Carbs 3%

Prep time: 15 minutes | Cook time: 45 minutes | Serves 4

FOr those who look for simplicity, strong taste, and few calories, this recipe offers you great taste, distinct flavor, and simplicity of preparation.

2 ounces (57 g) butter

2 pounds (907 g) chicken drumsticks

Salt and freshly ground black pepper, to taste

2 tablespoons olive oil

1 lemon, the juice

7 garlic cloves, sliced

½ cup fresh parsley, finely chopped

1. Start by preheating the oven to 450°F (235°C).
2. Grease the baking pan with butter and put the chicken drumsticks, season with salt and pepper generously.
3. Drizzle the olive oil and lemon juice over the chicken pieces. Sprinkle the garlic and parsley on top.
4. Bake the chicken for 30 to 40 minutes or until the garlic slices become golden and chicken pieces turn brown and roasted, the baking time may be longer if your drumsticks are on the large size. Lower the temperature considerably towards the end.

STORAGE: Low-carb garlic chicken can be stored covered in the fridge for 1 up to 4 days, it can even be kept in the freezer for 15 days.

REHEAT: Microwave, covered, until the desired temperature is reached or reheat in a frying pan or air fryer / instant pot, covered, on medium.

SERVE IT WITH: This wonderful recipe is served cold or hot, can be Serve with aioli and a hearty salad and toast with garlic. Some people favor it with a delectable cauliflower mash.

PER SERVING

calories: 542 | fat: 40.0g | total carbs: 4.0g | fiber: 1.0g | protein: 42.0g

Pie Keto Chicken Curry

Macros: Fat 84% | Protein 14% | Carbs 2%

Prep time:25 minutes | Cook time:40 minutes | Serves 4

Pie keto chicken curry is a popular recipe for children and adults, as it has a high nutritional value, this recipe is especially suitable for keto to preserve health and have i mentioned its distinctive taste? It is very suitable for family trips, too.

PIE CRUST:

¾ cup almond flour

4 tablespoons sesame seeds

4 tablespoons coconut flour

1 tablespoon ground psyllium husk powder

1 tablespoon baking powder

1 pinch salt

3 tablespoons olive oil or coconut oil

1 egg

4 tablespoons water

FILLING:

⅔ pound (302 g) cooked chicken

1 cup mayonnaise, keto-friendly

3 eggs

½ green bell pepper, finely chopped

1 teaspoon curry powder

½ teaspoon paprika powder

½ teaspoon onion powder

¼ teaspoon ground black pepper

4 ounces (113 g) cream cheese

5 ounces (142 g) shredded cheese

SPECIAL EQUIPMENT:

A 10-inch (25-cm) springform pan

1. Start by Preheating the oven to 350°F (180°C).
2. Place all the ingredients for the pie crust in a food processor for a couple of minutes until the dough firms into a ball. You can also mix the dough with a fork If you don't have a food processor.
3. Bring a springform pan with a diameter of no more than 10 inches (25 cm) (the spring form pan makes it easier to remove the pie when it is done). Attach a piece of parchment to the pan and grease the sides and bottom of the pan.
4. Spread the dough into the saucepan. Using your fingers or an oiled spatula. Pre-bake the crust for 10 to 15 minutes.
5. Mix together the other filling ingredients, and fill the pic crust. Bake for 35 to 40 minutes or until a good, golden brown has turned on the cookie.

STORAGE: The pie can be kept in the fridge for 2 days and in the freezer for a period not exceeding 3 months.

REHEAT: Microwave, covered, until the desired temperature is reached or reheat in a frying pan or air fryer / instant pot, covered, on medium.

SERVE IT WITH: The pie can be cut in medium size and served with hot sauce and vegetable salad for a great and delicious taste.

PER SERVING

calories: 1130 | fat: 105.0g | total carbs: 8.0g | fiber: 7.0g | protein: 39.0g

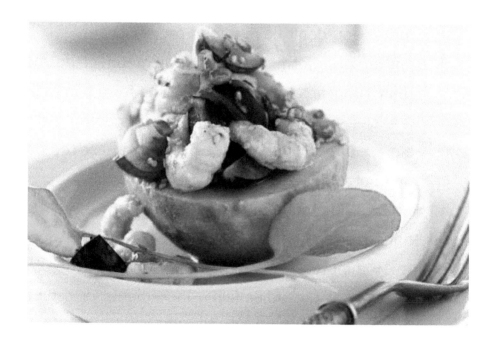

Chicken And Herb Butter with Keto Zucchini Roll-Ups

Macros: Fat 83% | Protein 13% | Carbs 4%

Prep time: 15 minutes | Cook time: 40 minutes | Serves 4

Chicken and herb butter with keto zucchini is the best recipe for a family gathering at dinner, where you find vitamins, protein, and calcium in one dish your child will enjoy a healthy and delicious meal as the family warms up .

ZUCCHINI ROLL-UPS:

1½ pounds (680 g) zucchini

½ teaspoon salt

3 ounces (85 g) butter

6 ounces (170 g) mushrooms, finely chopped

6 ounces (170 g) cream cheese

6 ounces (170 g) shredded Cheddar cheese

½ green bell pepper, chopped

2 ounces (57 g) air-dried chorizo, chopped

1 egg

1 teaspoon onion powder

2 tablespoons fresh parsley, chopped

½ teaspoon salt

¼ teaspoon pepper

CHICKEN:

4 (6-ounce / 170-g) chicken breasts

Salt and freshly ground pepper, to taste

1 ounce (28 g) butter, for frying

HERB BUTTER:

4 ounces (113 g) butter, at room temperature

1 garlic clove

½ teaspoon garlic powder

1 tablespoon fresh parsley, finely chopped

1 teaspoon lemon juice

½ teaspoon salt

1. Preheat the oven to 350°F (180°C). Cut the zucchini lengthwise into equal slices, half an inch, Pat dry with paper towels or a clean kitchen towel.and place it on a baking tray lined with parchment paper. Sprinkle salt on the zucchini and let stand for 10 minutes.

2. Bake for 20 minutes in the oven, or until the zucchini is tender. Transfer to a cooling rack from the oven, Dry more if needed.

3. Put the butter in the saucepan over medium heat, cut the mushrooms and put it in and stir fry well, let cool.

4. Add the remaining ingredients for the zucchini roll-ups to a bowl, except a third of the shredded cheese. Add the mushrooms and blend well.
5. Place a large amount of cheese on top of each zucchini slice.
6. Roll up and put it inside the baking dish with seams down, Sprinkle on top the remainder of the cheese.
7. Raise the temperature to 400°F (205°C). Bake for 20 minutes, or until the cheese turns bubbly and golden.
8. In the meantime, season your chicken and fry it over medium heat in butter until it is crispy on the outside and cooked through.

HERB BUTTER:
1. To prepare Herb butter mix the butter, garlic, garlic powder, fresh parsley, lemon juice, and salt. thoroughly in a small bowl.
2. Let sit for 30 minutes and serve on top of the chicken and zucchini roll-ups.

STORAGE: Store in an airtight container in the fridge for up to 5 days or in the freezer for up to 2 weeks.

REHEAT: Microwave, covered, until the desired temperature is reached or reheat in a frying pan.

SERVE IT WITH: Serve with a herb butter or keto-friendly mayonnaise and a green salad.

PER SERVING

calories: 913 | fat: 84.0g | total carbs: 10.0g | fiber: 3.0g | protein: 30.0g

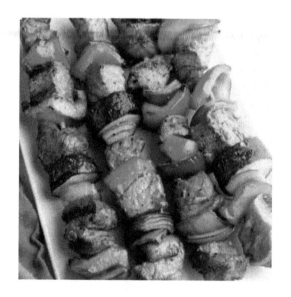

Keto Buffalo Drumsticks with Chili Aioli And Garlic

Macros: Fat 68% | Protein 30% | Carbs 2%

Prep time:10 minutes | Cook time:40 minutes | Serves 4

For those who love chicken with spices, peppers, and olive oil in an easy and simple way, and for those who work all day and want to enjoy a delicious meal, keto buffalo drumsticks with chili aioli and garlic is the best choice for fun and health. It's take 40 minutes to get ready. Cook it and enjoy the taste.

2 pounds (907 g) chicken drumsticks or chicken wings

CHILI AIOLI:

⅓ cup mayonnaise, keto-friendly

1 tablespoon smoked paprika powder or smoked chili powder

1 garlic clove, minced

2 tablespoons olive oil, and more for greasing the baking dish

2 tablespoons white wine vinegar

1 teaspoon salt

1 teaspoon paprika powder

1 tablespoon tabasco

1. Preheat the oven to 450°F (235°C).

2. Make the chili aioli: Combine the mayonnaise, smoked paprika powder, garlic clove, olive oil white wine vInegar, salt, paprika powder and tabasco for the marinade in a small bowl,

3. Put the drumsticks in a plastic bag, and pour the chili aioli into the plastic bag. Shake the bag thoroughly and let marinate for 10 minutes at room temperature.

4. Coat a baking dish with olive oil. Place the drumsticks in the baking dish and let bake in the preheated oven for 30 to 40 minutes or until they are done and have turned a nice color.

5. Remove the chicken wings from the oven and serve warm.

STORAGE: Store in an airtight container in the fridge for up to 3 days or in the freezer for week up to 1 month.

REHEAT: The chicken drumsticks or chicken wings with chili aioli, Can be heated with a frying pan, a microwave or grill easily.

SERVE IT WITH: serve with mayonnaise sauce, yogurt, and vegetable salad for a great and delicious taste.To make this a complete meal, serve the soup with crisp salad or roasted vegetables.

PER SERVING

calories: 570 | fat: 43.0g | total carbs: 3.0g | fiber: 1.0g | protein: 43.0g

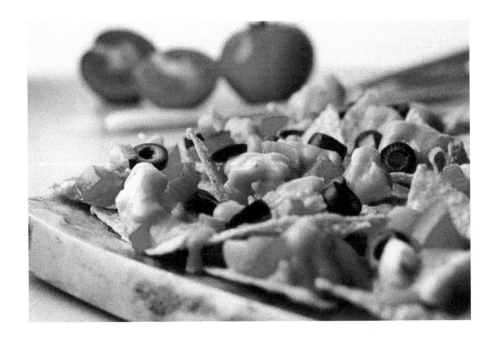

Coleslaw With Crunchy Keto Chicken Thighs

Macros: Fat 79% | Protein 19% | Carbs 2%

Prep time: 15 minutes | Cook time: 40 minutes | Serves 8

Who doesn't like coleslaw with crunchy keto chicken thighs? this recipe was really amazing, the marinade was very easy to make. It's one of my favorite keto dishes, it is so flavorful and all the ingredients are natural.

CHICKEN THIGHS:

1 teaspoon salt

½ cup sour cream

2 tablespoons jerk seasoning (cinnamon, paprika, tumeric, ginger, saffron and cumin)

2 pounds (907 g) chicken thighs

5 ounces (142 g) pork rinds

3 ounces (85 g) unsweetened shredded coconut

3 tablespoons olive oil

COLESLAW:

1 pound (454 g) green cabbage

1 cup mayonnaise, keto-friendly

Salt and freshly ground black pepper, to taste

SPECIAL EQUIPMENT:

2 big plastic bags

1. Preheat the oven to 350°F (180°C).

2. Mix together a marinade of jerk seasoning, salt and sour cream. And pour in a big plastic bag with the drumsticks, please keep the skin on the drumsticks.

3. Thoroughly shake and allow to marinate for 15 minutes.

4. Take the drumsticks out, and into a new, clean bag.

5. Put the pork rinds into a food processor and blend into fine crumbs, add in coconut flakes and blend a few more seconds.

6. Pour the pork mixture into the bag with the marinated chicken and shake.

7. Grease a baking dish, and put the chicken into it, drizzle with olive oil and bake for 40 to 50 minutes, or until the chicken is cooked through. Turn the drumsticks halfway through, if the breading has already turned a desirable golden brown color, lower the heat.

8. In the meantime, cut the cabbage finely with a sharp knife or with a mandolin or even a food processor. Put the coleslaw into a bowl, season with salt and pepper, and add mayonnaise, mix well and let sit for 10 minutes.

STORAGE: Store in an airtight container in the fridge for up to 5 days. You can freeze the chicken for 1 to 2 months, but can't freeze the coleslaw.

REHEAT: Microwave, covered or reheated in a frying pan until the desired temperature is reached.

SERVE IT WITH: To make this a complete meal, Serve the thighs chicken and the coleslaw with a glass of orange juice, enjoy!

PER SERVING

calories: 586 | fat: 51.2g | total carbs: 6.4g | fiber: 2.4g | protein: 27.2g

Gravy Bacon and Turkey
Macros: Fat 45% | Protein 53% | Carbs 2%

Prep time: 15 minutes | Cook time: 3 hours | Serves 14

This gravy bacon and turkey is very simple to make given that it is made in the same way conventional turkey gravy is made. One extra step is added when making the turkey, which sets this amazing gravy recipe apart!

To my family, it's one of our favorite dishes. I will show you in detail how to make turkey with bacon gravy here.

12 pounds (5.4 kg) turkey

Sea salt and fresh ground black pepper, to taste

1 pound (454 g) cherry tomatoes

1 cup red onions, diced

2 garlic cloves, minced

1 large celery stalk, diced

4 teaspoons fresh thyme, four small sprigs

8 ounces (227 g) bacon (10 slices, diced)

8 tablespoons butter

2 lemon, the juice

⅛ teaspoon guar gum (optional)

SPECIAL EQUIPMENT:

Kitchen twine

1. Start by preheating the oven to 350°F (180°C).

2. Remove the neck and giblets from the turkey, pat the turkey dry with paper towels and season both inside and outside of the turkey with salt and pepper.

3. Insert cherry tomatoes, onions, celery, garlic and thyme into the turkey cavity. Tie the legs together with kitchen twine, and put the turkey on a large roasting pan, tuck its wings under the body.

4. Cook the bacon in a large skillet over medium heat until crisp, for 7 to 8 minutes. Transfer to paper towels to drain, reserving the drippings in the skillet.

5. Add the ghee or butter to the skillet with the drippings and stir until melted, then pour into a bowl and stir in the lemon juice. Rub mixture all over the turkey.

6. Place into oven for 30 minutes. After every 30 minutes, baste the turkey with the drippings. Roast for about 3 hours or until a thermometer inserted into the thigh registers 165°F (74°C).

7. Remove from oven onto a serving tray to rest for at least 25 minutes before serving.

8. Meanwhile, pour the drippings into a saucepan. Whisk in the guar gum to thicken, after 2 minutes of whisking, add a touch more if you want a thicker gravy. Then add the reserved bacon for one amazing gravy.

STORAGE: Store in an airtight container in the fridge for up to 5 days. You can freeze the chicken for 1 to 2 months.

REHEAT: Microwave, covered or reheated in a frying pan until the desired temperature is reached.

SERVE IT WITH: Serve the dish with Antipasto Salad and a glass of juice!

PER SERVING calories: 693 | fat: 35.0g | total carbs: 3.7g | fiber: 0.7g | protein: 86.7g

Keto Chicken with Herb Butter
Macros: Fat 82% | Protein 17% | Carbs 1%

Prep time: 10 minutes | Cook time: 10 minutes | Serves 8

There is truly nothing better than a quick, delicious keto chicken with herb butter recipe that gets the dinner on the table in no time. Recipes for fast chicken breasts help me get the dinner on the table fast during the hectic weekends.

This 10-minute keto chicken with herb butter is a true gem and will become a family favorite.

HERB BUTTER:

6 ounces (170 g) herb butter, at room temperature

1 garlic clove, minced

½ teaspoon garlic powder

¼ cup fresh parsley, finely chopped

1 teaspoon lemon juice

½ teaspoon salt

FRIED CHICKEN:

3 tablespoons butter

4 chicken breasts

Salt and freshly ground black pepper, to taste

SERVING:

8 ounces (227 g) leafy greens (such as baby spinach)

1. Start with the herb butter. Mix the garlic, parsley, lemon juice and a pinch of salt thoroughly in a small bowl and let sit until it's time to serve.
2. Cut in half horizontally to make two thin chicken breasts so they cook evenly and quickly. Season the chicken with Italian seasoning, salt, pepper, and crushed red pepper.
3. Melt the butter over medium heat, in a large frying pan. Put in the chicken and fry in butter until the fillets are cooked through, or a meat thermometer inserted and registers 165°F (75°C). To prevent dry chicken fillets, lower the temperature toward the end.
4. Serve the chicken on a leafy greens bed and put a generous amount of herb butter over it.

STORAGE: Keep it in the fridge for up to 4 days or in the freezer for up to 1 month.

REHEAT: Reheat it until piping hot throughout. If you're using a microwave, be aware they do not heat evenly throughout, so take your food out halfway through cooking time and give it a stir.

SERVE IT WITH: To make this a complete meal, you can serve it with a side of pasta, veggies, or cauliflower rice.

PER SERVING

calories: 772 | fat: 70.3g | total carbs: 1.5g | fiber: 0.7g | protein. 34.1g

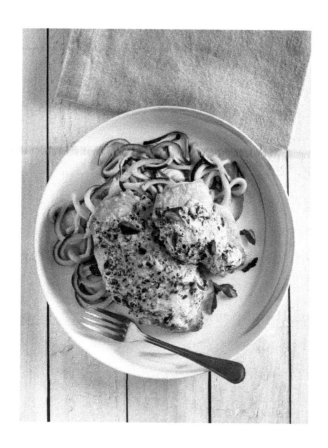

Chicken With Mushrooms and Parmesan Cheese

Macros: Fat 63% | Protein 33% | Carbs 4%

Prep time: 10 minutes | Cook time: 30 minutes | Serves 4

Chicken is always a favorite at week-night. This simple chicken with mushroom and Parmesan cheese features a creamy, cheesy mushroom sauce. It is a quick keto meal, ideal for busy evenings because it can be cooked and prepared in less than 30 minutes.

If you think you don't like mushrooms, think again, because this recipe is about to change the way you feel about mushrooms forever! And if you're already a fan of mushrooms like me and are looking for a way to uplift your game of mushroom-lovin dinner, this recipe has your name all over it.

2 tablespoons avocado oil

1½ pounds (680 g) boneless chicken thighs

Salt and freshly ground black pepper, to taste

4 garlic cloves, minced

8 ounces (227 g) cremini mushrooms, sliced

1½ cups heavy whipping cream

2 ounces (57 g) Parmesan cheese, grated

1 teaspoon fresh parsley

1. Heat the avocado oil in a large skillet over medium heat. Season the chicken thighs with salt and pepper. Fry in the skillet until browned or cooked; remove the chicken to a slotted spoon plate, conserve the juices in the pan.
2. Add garlic to the frying pan and stir-fry until soft; add mushrooms and sauté for around 5 to 7 minutes, until softened.
3. Put heavy cream on low heat, and stir well. Stirring frequently for about 10 minutes, allow to simmer, incorporate Parmesan cheese to melt. Add salt and chili pepper to taste.
4. Return the chicken to the skillet and garnish with sauce. Serve with parsley.

STORAGE: Keep a stash of lidded containers so that you have something to store your leftovers in. Use freezer bags if you don't have space to store a lot of containers. Keep it in the fridge for up to 2 to 3 days or in the freezer for up to 3 weeks.

REHEAT: Microwave, covered, or reheated in a frying pan or instant pot, covered, on medium until the desired temperature is reached.

SERVE IT WITH: Serve with a fresh side salad or steamed low-carb vegetables like broccoli, spinach, or asparagus.

PER SERVING

calories: 584 | fat: 41.0g | total carbs: 6.0g | fiber: 0.6g | protein: 48.4g

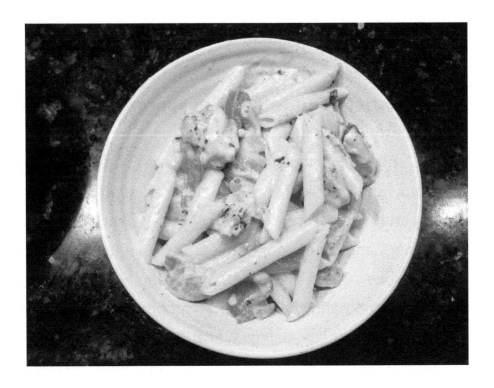

Sausage & Turnip Soup
Ingredients for 4 servings

3 turnips, chopped

2 celery sticks, chopped

2 tbsp butter

1 tbsp olive oil

1 pork sausage, sliced

2 cups vegetable broth

½ cup sour cream

3 green onions, chopped

Salt and black pepper, to taste

Directions and Total Time: approx. 40 minutes

Sauté green onions in melted butter over medium heat until soft and golden, about 3 minutes. Add celery and turnip, and cook for another 5 minutes. Pour the vegetable broth and 2 cups of water over. Bring to a simmer and cook for about 20 minutes until the vegetables are tender. Remove from heat. Puree the soup with a hand blender until smooth. Add sour cream and adjust the seasoning. Warm the olive oil in a skillet. Add the pork sausage and cook for 5 minutes. Serve the soup topped with pork sausage.

Per serving: Cal 275; Fat 23.1g; Net Carbs 6.g; Protein 7.4g

Cauliflower Cheese Soup
Ingredients for 4 servings

½ head cauliflower, chopped

2 tbsp coconut oil

½ cup leeks, chopped

1 celery stalk, chopped

1 serrano pepper, chopped

1 tsp garlic puree

1 ½ tbsp flaxseed meal

1 ½ cups coconut milk

6 oz Monterey Jack, shredded

Salt and black pepper, to taste

Fresh parsley, chopped

Directions and Total Time: approx. 25 minutes

In a deep pan over medium heat, melt the coconut oil and sauté the serrano pepper, celery, and leeks until soft, about 5 minutes. Add in coconut milk, garlic puree, cauliflower, 2 cups of water, and flaxseed meal.

While covered partially, allow simmering for 10 minutes or until cooked through. Whizz with an immersion blender until smooth. Fold in the shredded cheese, and stir to ensure the cheese is completely melted and you have a homogenous mixture. Season with pepper and salt to taste. Decorate with parsley and serve warm.

Per serving: Cal 312, Fat 16g, Net Carbs 7.1g, Protein 13g

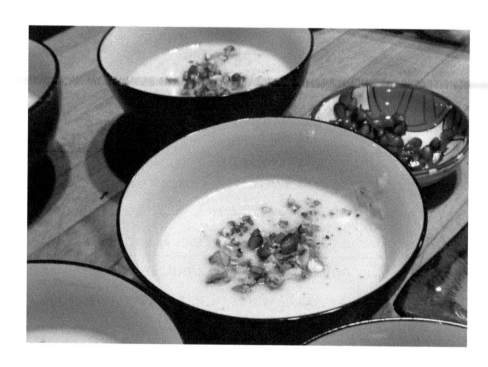

Cheese Cream Soup with Chicken

Ingredients for 4 servings

2 cups cooked and shredded chicken

1 carrot, chopped

1 onion, chopped

3 tbsp butter

4 cups chicken broth

2 tbsp cilantro, chopped

1/3 cup buffalo sauce

½ cup cream cheese

Salt and black pepper, to taste

Directions and Total Time: approx. 20 minutes

In a skillet over medium heat, warm butter and sauté carrot and onion until tender, about 5 minutes. Add the chicken and broth and heat until hot but do not bring to a boil. Season with salt and pepper. Stir in buffalo sauce and cream cheese and cook until heated through, about 2-3 minutes Serve garnished with cilantro.

Per serving: Cal 487; Fat 41g; Net Carbs 7.2g; Protein 16g

Cheesy Chicken Soup with Spinach
Ingredients for 4 servings

2 tbsp olive oil

1 onion, chopped

2 garlic cloves, minced

1 carrot, chopped

1 celery stalk, chopped

1 chicken breast, cubed

1 cup spinach

4 cups chicken broth

1 cup cheddar, shredded

½ tsp chili powder

½ tsp ground cumin

Salt and black pepper, to taste

Directions and Total Time: approx. 45 minutes

Warm the olive oil in a pot over medium heat and sauté chicken for 2-3 minutes. Add and stir-fry the onion, garlic, celery, and carrot for 5 minutes or until the vegetables are tender. Season with chili powder, cumin, salt, and pepper. Add the chicken broth and bring to a boil; cook for 15-20 minutes. Stir in in spinach and cook for 5-6 minutes until wilted. Top with cheddar cheese.

Per serving: Cal 351; Fat 22g; Net Carbs 4.3g; Protein 22g

Zucchini & Leek Turkey Soup

Ingredients for 4 servings

2 cups turkey meat, cooked and choppe d

1 onion, chopped

1 garlic clove, minced

3 celery stalks, chopped

2 leeks, chopped

2 tbsp butter

4 cups chicken stock

Salt and black pepper, to taste

¼ cup fresh parsley, chopped

1 large zucchini, spiralized

Directions and Total Time: approx. 40 minutes

Melt the butter in a pot over medium heat. Place the leeks, celery, onion, and garlic and cook for 5 minutes. Add in the turkey meat, black pepper, salt, and stock, and cook for 20 minutes. Stir in the zucchini and cook for 5 minutes. Serve in bowls sprinkled with parsley.

Per serving: Cal 312; Fat 13g; Net Carbs 4.3g; Protein 16g

Tomato Soup with Parmesan Croutons
Ingredients for 6 servings

Parmesan Croutons

4 tbsp butter, softened

4 tbsp grated Parmesan

3 egg whites

1 ¼ cups almond flour

2 tsp baking powder

5 tbsp psyllium husk powder

Tomato Soup

3 tbsp olive oil

2 lb fresh ripe tomatoes

4 cloves garlic, peeled only

1 small white onion, diced

1 red bell pepper, diced

1 cup coconut cream

½ tsp dried rosemary

½ tsp dried oregano

Salt and black pepper to taste

Directions and **Total Time: approx. 1 hour 25 minutes**

Preheat oven to 350 F. Line a baking sheet with wax paper. In a bowl, combine almond flour, baking powder, and psyllium husk powder. Mix in the egg whites. Whisk

72

for 30 seconds until combined but not overly mixed. Form 8 flat pieces out of the dough. Place on the baking sheet while leaving enough room between each to allow rising. Bake for 30 minutes. Let the croutons cool. Break into halves. Mix the butter with Parmesan cheese. Spread the mixture in the inner parts of the croutons. Bake for 5 minutes.

In a baking dish, add tomatoes, garlic, onion, bell pepper, and drizzle with olive oil. Roast vegetables in the oven for 25 minutes and after broil for 4 minutes. Transfer to a blender and add in coconut cream, rosemary, oregano, salt, and pepper. Puree until smooth. Top with croutons.

Per serving: Cal 429; Fat 41g; Net Carbs 6g; Protein 11g

Creamy Coconut Soup with Chicken
Ingredients for 4 servings

3 tbsp butter

1 onion, chopped

2 chicken breasts, chopped

Salt and black pepper, to taste

½ cup coconut cream

¼ cup celery, chopped

Directions and Total Time: approx. 25 minutes

Warm the butter in a pot over medium heat. Sauté the onion and celery for 3 minutes until tender. Stir in chicken, 4 cups of water, salt, and pepper. Cook for 15 minutes. Stir in coconut cream. Serve warm.

Per serving: Cal 394; Fat 24g; Net Carbs 6.1g; Protein 29g

Cream of Cauliflower & Leek Soup

Ingredients for 4 servings

4 cups vegetable broth

16 oz cauliflower florets

1 celery stalk, chopped

1 onion, chopped

1 cup leeks, chopped

2 tbsp butter

1 tbsp olive oil

1 cup heavy cream

½ tsp red pepper flakes

Directions and Total Time: approx. 45 minutes

Warm butter and olive oil in a pot set over medium heat and sauté onion, leeks, and celery for 5 minutes. Stir in the broth and cauliflower and bring to a boil; simmer for 30 minutes. Transfer the mixture to an immersion blender and puree; add in the heavy cream and stir. Decorate with red pepper flakes and serve.

Per serving: Cal 255; Fat 21g; Net Carbs 5.3g; Protein 4.4g

Broccoli & Spinach Soup

Ingredients for 4 servings

2 tbsp butter

1 onion, chopped

1 garlic clove, minced

2 heads broccoli, cut in florets

2 stalks celery, chopped

4 cups vegetable broth

1 cup baby spinach

Salt and black pepper to taste

1 tbsp basil, chopped

Parmesan, shaved to serve

Directions and Total Time: approx. 25 minutes

Melt the butter in a saucepan over medium heat. Sauté the garlic and onion for 3 minutes until softened. Mix in the broccoli and celery and cook for 4 minutes until slightly tender. Pour in the broth, bring to a boil, then reduce the heat to medium-low, and simmer covered for about 5 minutes.

Drop in the spinach to wilt, adjust the seasonings, and cook for 4 minutes. Ladle soup into serving bowls. Serve with a sprinkle of grated Parmesan cheese and basil.

Per serving: Cal 123; Fat 11g; Net Carbs 3.2g; Protein 1.8g

Cream of Roasted Jalapeño Soup

Ingredients for 4 servings

2 tbsp melted butter

1 jalapeño pepper, halved

6 green bell peppers, halved

1 bulb garlic, halved, not peeled

6 tomatoes, halved

3 cups vegetable broth

½ cup heavy cream

3 tbsp grated Parmesan

2 tbsp chopped chives

Salt and black pepper to taste

Directions and Total Time: approx. 45 min + cooling time

Preheat oven to 350 F. Arrange bell peppers, jalapeño pepper, and garlic on a baking pan and roast for 15 minutes. Add in tomatoes and roast for 15 minutes. Let cool. Peel the skins and place them in a blender.

Add salt, pepper, butter, vegetable broth, and heavy cream; puree until smooth. Transfer to a pot over medium heat and cook for 3-4 minutes. Serve into bowls sprinkled with Parmesan cheese and chives.

Per serving: Cal 191; Net Carbs 8.7g; Fat 9g; Protein 5.3g

Creamy Chicken And Ham Meatballs
Macros: Fat: 76% | Protein: 21% | Carbs: 3%

Prep time: 30 minutes | Cook time: 15 minutes | Serves 6

Meatballs are a delicious addition to every meal. From simple dishes to complex ones, this delicious meatball dish can be served alone or can be the perfect addition to every meal. These meatballs will come out juicy and are perfect for family dinners and parties. Grab a fork and dive in.

1 pound (454 g) ground chicken

⅓ cup blanched almond flour

½ teaspoon onion powder

1 egg, lightly beaten

½ teaspoon salt

½ teaspoon garlic powder

6 ounces (170 g) ham steak, cubed into 20 even pieces

1 tablespoon olive oil

1 tablespoon butter

¾ cup chicken broth

1 teaspoon Dijon mustard

½ cup heavy cream

1 cup shredded Swiss cheese

Freshly ground black pepper, to taste

2 tablespoons minced fresh parsley

1. Mix the chicken with the almond flour, onion powder, egg, salt, and garlic powder in a bowl. Roll a cube of ham into a 1½-inch ball with the chicken around it and put it on a plate. Make 20 chicken-covered ham meatballs from this mixture.

2. Heat the olive oil in a nonstick skillet over medium-high heat. Arrange the meatballs in the skillet and cook for 3 minutes or until lightly browned. Flip them and cook for another 3 to 4 minutes, then remove them from the skillet to a plate.

3. Reduce the heat to medium and add the butter to melt. Mix in the chicken broth and the mustard, then simmer for about 3 minutes.

4. Mix in the cream and Swiss cheese until it has completely melted, then put the meatballs back into the skillet. Let it cook for 3 to 4 minutes or until the sauce reduces in half.

5. Sprinkle with black pepper and parsley, then serve hot.

STORAGE: Store in an airtight container in the fridge for up to 4 days or in the freezer for up to 1 month.

REHEAT: Microwave, covered, until the desired temperature is reached or reheat in a frying pan or air fryer / instant pot, covered, on medium.

SERVE IT WITH: To make this a complete meal, serve it with mushroom and cauliflower salad.

PER SERVING

calories: 544 | fat: 45.9g | total carbs: 4.7g | fiber: 0.5g | protein: 28.4g

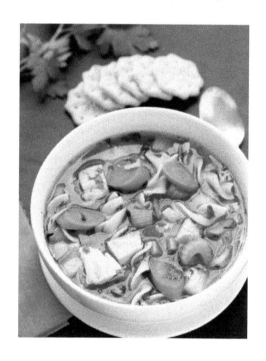

Buttery Chicken and Mushrooms

Macros: Fat: 56% | Protein: 36% | Carbs: 8%

Prep time: 10 minutes | Cook time: 30 minutes | Serves 4

This delicious chicken and mushroom dish is a quick and easy dish to make. Whether during busy weekdays or for want of a variety, this low-carb dish is the way to go. It is perfect for parties and family gatherings.

2 boneless chicken breasts, skin-on

Salt and ground black pepper, to taste

2 tablespoons olive oil

8 ounces (227 g) fresh mushrooms, cut into ¼ -inch-thick slices

½ cup of water

1 tablespoon butter

1. Start by preheating the oven to 400°F (205°C).

2. On a plate, sprinkle salt and pepper over the chicken.

3. Heat the olive oil in a frying pan over medium-high heat. Add the chicken breasts, skin side down, and cook for 5 minutes or until browned.

4. Flip the chicken and add the mushrooms. Sprinkle salt over the mushrooms and cook for 5 minutes, stirring occasionally, or until the mushrooms shrink slightly.

5. Remove the pan from the heat and put it into the oven. Bake for 15 to 20 minutes or until a meat thermometer inserted in the center of the chicken reads at least 165ºF (74ºC).

6. Remove the chicken from the oven and put it on a plate. Cover the plate loosely with a foil and set aside.

7. Put the pan over medium-high heat and cook the mushrooms for 5 minutes until the bottom of the pan starts to brown. Pour the water into the pan and use a spatula or a wooden spoon to scrape up the bits. Cook for 2 minutes or until the water has reduced by half.

STORAGE: Store in an airtight container in the fridge for up to 4 days or in the freezer for up to 1 month.

REHEAT: Microwave, covered, until the desired temperature is reached or reheat in a frying pan or instant pot, covered, on medium.

SERVE IT WITH: To make this a complete meal, serve it on a bed of zucchini noodles.

PER SERVING

calories: 368 | fat: 23.2g | total carbs: 8.5g | fiber: 1.3g | protein: 31.2g

Sour Pepper Chicken

Macros: Fat: 46% | Protein: 51% | Carbs: 3%

Prep time: 15 minutes | Cook time: 20 minutes | Serves 6

This grilled sour pepper chicken wakes up every taste bud with its distinguishing taste. It has a crunchy, grilled skin with a perfectly-spiced, juicy, tender meat that leaves you wanting more. This dish is quick and easy to make which makes it a perfect dinner for busy weekdays.

1 teaspoon freshly ground black pepper

½ cup lemon juice

¼ cup olive oil

1 tablespoon distilled white vinegar

6 cloves garlic, crushed or very finely minced

2 tablespoons dried oregano

1 teaspoon red pepper flakes, to taste

6 chicken leg quarters

Kosher salt, to taste

1 lemon, cut into wedges

1. In a large bowl, whisk the black pepper, lemon juice, oil, vinegar, garlic, oregano, and red pepper flakes together.
2. Cut 2 deep slices into each chicken leg, making sure that it reaches the bone, then sprinkle generously

with the kosher salt and dunk them into the bowl of mixture. Wrap the bowl in plastic and put in the refrigerator to marinate for 4 to 12 hours.

3. Preheat the grill to medium-high heat.
4. Discard the marinade and pat dry the chicken legs with paper towels.
5. Put the chicken leg on the grill, skin side down, and cook for 6 to 7 minutes on each side or until the juices run clear and no pink. Cook for another 8 minutes or until cooked through.
6. Remove the chicken legs from the grill and serve them on a plate, and squeeze the lemon wedges over.

STORAGE: Store in an airtight container in the fridge for up to 4 days or in the freezer for up to 1 month.

REHEAT: Microwave, covered, until the desired temperature is reached or reheat in a frying pan or air fryer / instant pot, covered, on medium.

SERVE IT WITH: To make this a complete meal, serve it with a glass of sparkling water.

PER SERVING

calories: 402 | fat: 20.4g | total carbs: 4.4g | fiber: 1.0g | protein: 51.3g

Italian Garlic Chicken Kebab

Macros: Fat: 35% | Protein: 63% | Carbs: 2%

Prep time: 20 minutes | Cook time: 15 minutes | Serves 8

This dish is the perfect go-to for everyone. It is a crowd-pleaser in every party, gathering, brunch, or just a simple dinner. It freezes and reheats well which means that you can get your favorite dish anytime, anywhere.

¼ cup coconut aminos

¼ teaspoon onion powder

2 tablespoons lemon juice

4 tablespoons olive oil, divided

¾ teaspoon Italian seasoning

3 tablespoons dry white wine

1 clove garlic, crushed

1 teaspoon grated fresh ginger root

1 pinch ground black pepper

8 skinless, boneless chicken breasts, cut into strips

SPECIAL EQUIPMENT:

8 skewers, soaked for at least 30 minutes to avoid burning during grilling

1. Put the coconut aminos, onion powder, lemon juice, 2 tablespoons of olive oil, Italian seasoning, dry white wine, garlic, ginger root, and black pepper in a Ziploc

bag and mix them together. Put the chicken in the bag. Shake the bag to make sure the chicken is coated in the spices, then seal the bag and put it in the refrigerator to marinate for 3 hours.

2. Preheat an outdoor grill to medium-high heat.

3. Run each of the skewers through the chicken strips and set aside. Pour the marinade into a pan over high heat and let it boil.

4. Brush the preheated grill grates with 1 tablespoon of olive oil and place the chicken skewers on the grates to grill for 16 minutes. Brush the chicken skewers with the remaining olive oil and flip halfway through the cooking time. Cover the chicken with the sauce generously as it grills.

5. When the chicken juices run clear, remove it from the grill, and serve on a plate.

STORAGE: Store in an airtight container in the fridge for up to 4 days or in the freezer for up to 1 month.

REHEAT: Microwave, covered, until the desired temperature is reached or reheat in a frying pan or air fryer / instant pot, covered, on medium.

SERVE IT WITH: To make this a complete meal, serve it with cheesy broccoli salad.

PER SERVING

calories: 339 | fat: 13.0g | total carbs: 2.4g | fiber: 0.1g | protein: 53.2g

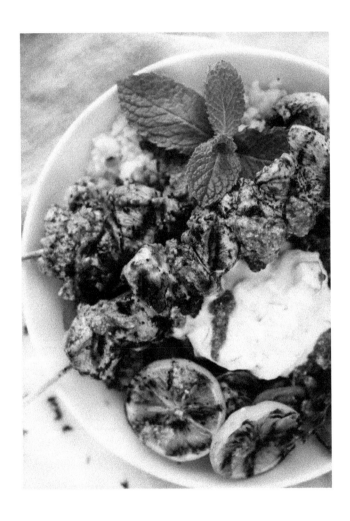

Chicken In Tomatoes and Herbs

Macros: Fat: 28% | Protein: 65% | Carbs: 7%

Prep time: 10 minutes | Cook time: 25 minutes | Serves 6

This herb chicken dish will become your favorite go-to recipe for every occasion. It is the perfect way to add a juicy chicken to salads, wraps, pasta, and any other dish. Perfect for kids and adults, any event with this dish will be fondly remembered.

6 skinless, boneless chicken breasts

1 teaspoon garlic salt

Freshly ground black pepper, to taste

2 tablespoons olive oil

1 onion, thinly sliced

1 (14½-ounce / 411-g) can diced tomatoes

½ cup balsamic vinegar

HERBS:

1 teaspoon dried basil

1 teaspoon dried oregano

1 teaspoon dried rosemary

½ teaspoon dried thyme

1. Sprinkle all sides of the chicken with garlic salt and pepper.

2. Pour the olive oil into the pan over medium heat and brown the chicken breasts in the pan for 3 to 4 minutes on each side. Mix in the onions and cook for 3 o 4 minutes until it is browned.

3. Pour the tomatoes and vinegar over the chicken then season with the herbs. Cook on low heat for 15 minutes until the juices are clear.

4. Remove them from the heat and serve on a plate.

STORAGE: Store in an airtight container in the fridge for up to 4 days or in the freezer for up to 1 month.

REHEAT: Microwave, covered, until the desired temperature is reached or reheat in a frying pan or air fryer / instant pot, covered, on medium.

SERVE IT WITH: To make this a complete meal, serve it with a bowl of green salad.

PER SERVING

calories: 356 | fat: 10.9g | total carbs: 6.6g | fiber: 1.6g | protein: 53.9g

Air-Fried Garlic-Lemon Chicken

Macros: Fat: 70% | Protein: 27% | Carbs: 3%

Prep time: 10 minutes | Cook time: 25 minutes | Serves 4

This deliciously crunchy chicken thigh dish is in a league of its own. Air fried with the best ingredients to bring out its flavor, every bite will explode in mouth-watering goodness that will overwhelm your senses and have you reaching for more.

¼ cup lemon juice

2 cloves garlic, minced

¼ teaspoon salt

⅛ teaspoon ground black pepper

2 tablespoons olive oil

1 teaspoon Dijon mustard

4 skin-on, bone-in chicken thighs

4 lemon wedges

1. In a bowl, mix the lemon juice, garlic, salt, black pepper, olive oil, and mustard together. Set aside.
2. Put the chicken thighs into a Ziploc bag and pour the marinade in. Make sure that the chicken thighs are well coated in the marinade, then seal the bag and put it in the refrigerator for at least 2 hours.
3. Preheat the air fryer to 375°F (190°C).

4. Remove the chicken from the marinade and dry it with paper towels.

5. Put the chicken in the air fryer basket and fry in batches for 22 to 24 minutes or until the juices are clear and a meat thermometer should read 165°F (74°C). Flip the chicken thighs halfway through the cooking time.

6. Transfer the chicken to a plate and squeeze the lemon wedges over, then serve.

STORAGE: Store in an airtight container in the fridge for up to 4 days or in the freezer for up to 1 month.

REHEAT: Microwave, covered, until the desired temperature is reached or reheat in a frying pan or air fryer / instant pot, covered, on medium.

SERVE IT WITH: To make this a complete meal, you can serve it with stir-fried zoodles.

PER SERVING

calories: 503 | fat: 39.0g | total carbs: 5.5g | fiber: 0.3g | protein: 32.3g

Spicy Burnt-Fried Chicken

Macros: Fat: 27% | Protein: 71% | Carbs: 2%

Prep time: 10 minutes | Cook time: 20 minutes |

Serves 2

You cannot deny that a slightly burnt or blackened taste gives any chicken an extra kick. This delicious burnt-fried chicken is guaranteed to leave you wanting some more. Generously coated in hot spices, it is the perfect meal to kick out the cold and delight your taste buds.

½ teaspoon cayenne pepper

½ teaspoon onion powder

½ teaspoon black pepper

2 teaspoons paprika

1 teaspoon ground thyme

1 teaspoon cumin

¼ teaspoon salt

2 (12-ounce / 340-g) skinless, boneless chicken breasts

2 teaspoons olive oil

1. Mix the cayenne pepper, onion powder, black pepper, paprika, thyme, cumin, and salt in a bowl.

2. Rub the chicken breasts with the olive oil, then put it in the spice mixture. Make sure they are coated all around with the spices, then set aside to marinate for 5 minutes.

3. Preheat the air fryer to 375°F (190°C).

4. Put the chicken in the air fryer basket and cook for 10 minutes. Flip it over and cook for another 10 minutes.

5. Remove the chicken from the basket to a plate and let it rest for 5 minutes before serving.

STORAGE: Store in an airtight container in the fridge for up to 4 days or in the freezer for up to 1 month.

REHEAT: Microwave, covered, until the desired temperature is reached or reheat in a frying pan or air fryer / instant pot, covered, on medium.

SERVE IT WITH: To make this a complete meal, serve it with mashed cauliflower.

PER SERVING

calories: 464 | fat: 14.1g | total carbs: 3.0g | fiber: 1.4g | protein: 77.3g

Crunchy Taco Chicken Wings

Macros: Fat: 28% | Protein: 71% | Carbs: 1%

Prep time: 5 minutes | Cook time: 15 minutes | Serves 5

Take the taste of that crunchy taco you absolutely love and put it on these chicken wings dish. This dish is a quick and easy dish that promises to take your taste buds on an amazing ride. From the crunchy, well-seasoned chicken back to the soft and spicy meat, this chicken dish will always make a reappearance on your table.

3 pounds (1.4 kg) chicken wings

1 tablespoon taco seasoning mix

2 teaspoons olive oil

1. Put the chicken wings in a Ziploc bag, then add the taco seasoning and olive oil.
2. Seal the bag and shake well until the chicken is coated thoroughly.
3. Preheat the air fryer to 350°F (180°C).
4. Put the chicken in the air fryer basket and cook for 6 minutes on each side until crispy.
5. Remove the chicken from the basket and serve on a plate.

STORAGE: Store in an airtight container in the fridge for up to 4 days or in the freezer for up to 1 month.

REHEAT: Microwave, covered, until the desired temperature is reached or reheat in a frying pan or air fryer / instant pot, covered, on medium.

SERVE IT WITH: To make this a complete meal, serve it with a bowl of cauliflower rice and a glass of sparkling water.

PER SERVING

calories: 364 | fat: 11.4g | total carbs: 1.0g | fiber: 0.2g | protein: 59.9g

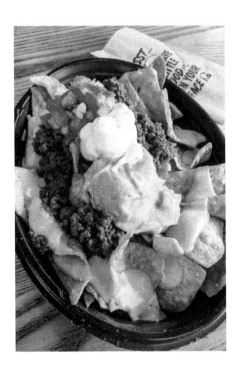

Spicy Cheesy Stuffed Avocados

Macros: Fat: 63% | Protein: 24% | Carbs: 12%

Prep time: 10 minutes | Cook time: 8 minutes | Serves 8

Perfect for brunch and parties with kids and adults, this dish is a healthy, low-carb healthy alternative to unhealthy snacks. Each bite is loaded with the delicious, healthy avocado which is the perfect ingredients for every low-carb diet.

4 avocados, halved and pitted

2 cooked chicken breasts, shredded

4 ounces (113 g) cream cheese, softened

¼ teaspoon ground black pepper

1 pinch cayenne pepper

¼ cup tomatoes, chopped

¼ teaspoon salt

½ cup shredded Parmesan cheese, or more to taste

SPECIAL EQUIPMENT:

8 muffin cups, for stabilizing the avocado halves

1. Start by preheating the oven to 400°F (205°C)
2. Spoon some of the avocado flesh in a bowl. Add the chicken, cream cheese, black pepper, cayenne pepper, tomatoes, and salt to the bowl and mix well.

Spoon the mixture into each of the avocado wells then top it with a layer of Parmesan cheese.

3. Put the avocado halves in muffin cups, facing up, to stabilize them.

4. Put the cups in the preheated oven to bake for 8 to 10 minutes, or until the cheese is melted.

5. Remove them from the oven and serve hot.

STORAGE: Store in an airtight container in the fridge for up to 4 days or in the freezer for up to 1 month.

REHEAT: Microwave, covered, until the desired temperature is reached or reheat in a frying pan or air fryer / instant pot, covered, on medium.

SERVE IT WITH: To make this a complete meal, serve it with jicama and daikon radish salad with a glass of sparkling water.

PER SERVING

calories: 308 | fat: 22.9g | total carbs: 10.3g | fiber: 6.8g | protein: 18.0g

Crispy Keto Wings with Rich Broccoli
Macros: Fat 61% | Protein 34% | Carbs 5%

Prep time:15 minutes | Cook time: 45 minutes | Serves 6

The crispness and fragrance of this tender chicken wings will catch your palate, and served with tiny broccoli florets to help balance the rich, creaminess of the dish. It's is a match made in heaven.

BAKED CHICKEN WINGS:

½ lemon, juice and zest

2 teaspoons ground ginger

¼ teaspoon cayenne pepper

¼ cup olive oil

1 teaspoon salt

3 pounds (1.4 kg) chicken wings

CREAMY BROCCOLI:

1½ pounds (680 g) broccoli, cut into florets

¼ cup chopped fresh dill

1 cup mayonnaise, keto-friendly

Salt and freshly ground black pepper, to taste

1. Preheat the oven to 400°F (205°C).

2. Combine the lemon juice, lemon zest, ground ginger, cayenne pepper, olive oil, and salt in a Ziploc bag,

then put the chicken wings in the bag. Shake to coat well.

3. Arrange the bag in the refrigerator to marinate for at least 45 minutes.

4. Arrange the well-coated chicken wings in a lightly greased baking dish. PLace the dish in the preheated oven.

5. Bake for 45 minutes, or until no pink and the juice of the chicken wings run clear.

6. Meanwhile, blanch the broccoli in a pot of salted water for 5 minutes or until lightly softened.

7. Transfer the broccoli to a large bowl, and add the remaining ingredients. Toss to combine well.

8. Serve the baked chicken wings with creamy broccoli aside.

STORAGE: Store in an airtight container in the fridge for up to 4 days.

REHEAT: Microwave, covered, until the desired temperature is reached or reheat in a frying pan or air fryer / instant pot, covered, on medium.

SERVE IT WITH: To make this a complete meal, you can serve it with mushroom and salmon salad, and strawberry smoothie.

PER SERVING

calories: 657 | fat: 44.9g | total carbs: 8.5g | fiber: 3.1g | protein: 53.5g

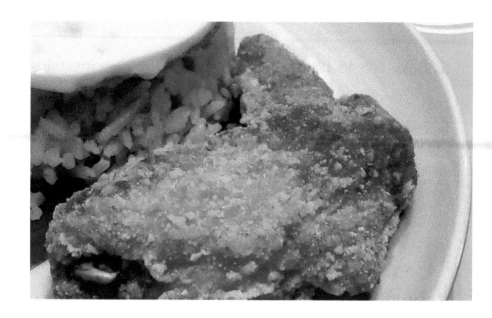

Spicy Oven-Baked Chicken

Macros: Fat: 21% | Protein: 74% | Carbs: 5%

Prep time: 10 minutes | Cook time: 20 minutes | Serves 8

This spicy oven-baked chicken is the perfect highlight of every gathering. It is a juicy dish that is perfect for salads, wraps, pasta, and any sandwiches of your choice. It has a delicious crispy skin with soft and juicy meat that makes each bite a pleasure.

1 teaspoon dried thyme

1 teaspoon white pepper

½ teaspoon cayenne pepper

4 teaspoons salt

2 teaspoons paprika

1 teaspoon onion powder

½ teaspoon black pepper

½ teaspoon garlic powder

2 onions, quartered

2 (4-pound / 1.8-kg) whole chickens, giblets removed, rinsed and drained

1. Mix the thyme, white pepper, cayenne, salt, paprika, onion powder, black pepper, and garlic powder in a bowl.

2. Coat the inside of the chicken and the outer part with the spice mixture, then put 1 onion inside the chicken.

3. Put the chicken in a Ziploc bag and seal it. Place the chicken in a refrigerator for 4 to 6 hours, preferably overnight.

4. Preheat the oven to 40 0 °F (20 5 °C) .

5. Remove the chicken from the bag and put it in a roasting pan. Put the pan in the oven to bake for about 20 minutes, or until an instant-read thermometer inserted into the thickest part registers at least 16 5°F (7 4°C).

6. Remove the chicken from the oven. Let it rest for 10 minutes before slicing to serve.

STORAGE: Store in an airtight container in the fridge for up to 4 days or in the freezer for up to 1 month.

REHEAT: Microwave, covered, until the desired temperature is reached or reheat in a frying pan or air fryer / instant pot, covered, on medium.

SERVE IT WITH: To make this a complete meal, serve it with a bowl of green salad.

PER SERVING

calories: 268 | fat: 6.3g | total carbs: 3.7g | fiber: 0.9g | protein: 46.6g

Buttery Cheesy Garlic Chicken

Macros: Fat: 46% | Protein: 51% | Carbs: 3%

Prep time: 15 minutes | Cook time: 40 minutes | Serves 8

This buttery cheesy garlic chicken dish is perfectly cooked for all occasions. It is easy to make with ingredients you probably have at home. This recipe is going to be a constant request from family and friends during any parties.

½ cup butter

4 cloves garlic, minced

1½ cups shredded Cheddar cheese

¼ teaspoon dried parsley

¼ teaspoon dried oregano

¼ cup coconut flour

½ cup freshly grated Parmesan cheese

¼ teaspoon ground black pepper

⅛ teaspoon salt

8 skinless, boneless chicken breasts, pounded thin

1. Start by preheating the oven to 350°F (180°C).
2. Put the butter in a pan and melt over low heat. Add the garlic to cook for 3 minutes or until lightly browned. Transfer the garlic butter to a bowl. Set aside.

3. Mix the Cheddar cheese, parsley, oregano, coconut flour, Parmesan cheese, black pepper, and salt together in a separate bowl.

4. Dredge each chicken breast into the garlic butter, then coat it with the cheese mixture.

5. Place the chicken breasts on a baking dish and pour the remaining garlic butter and cheese mixture over them, then put the baking dish in the preheated oven.

6. Bake for 30 minutes until an instant-read thermometer inserted in the center of the chicken register at least 165ºF (74ºC).

7. Remove the chicken from the oven and serve warm.

STORAGE: Store in an airtight container in the fridge for up to 4 days or in the freezer for up to 1 month.

REHEAT: Microwave, covered, until the desired temperature is reached or reheat in a frying pan or air fryer / instant pot, covered, on medium.

SERVE IT WITH: To make this a complete meal, serve it with a bowl of green salad.

PER SERVING

calories: 506 | fat: 26.3g | total carbs: 2.9g | fiber: 0.1g | protein: 61.3g

Pan-Fried Creamy Chicken with Tarragon

Macros: Fat: 41% | Protein: 58% | Carbs: 1%

Prep time: 15 minutes | Cook time: 30 minutes | Serves 4

This pan-fried chicken dish is creamy and delicious. Made with mustard and fresh tarragon, this low-carb dish will hit you with a hint of spice and flavor with the buttery juiciness of the chicken.

1 tablespoon butter

1 tablespoon olive oil

4 skinless, boneless chicken breasts

Salt and fleshly ground black pepper, to taste

½ cup heavy cream

1 tablespoon Dijon mustard

2 teaspoons chopped fresh tarragon

1. Melt the butter in a pan over medium-high heat, then add the olive oil.

2. Season the chicken with salt and pepper then put it in the pan to fry for 15 minutes on both sides until the juices are clear. Remove them from the pan and set aside.

3. Pour the heavy cream in the pan and use a wooden spoon to scrape the parts stuck to the pan, then add

the mustard and the tarragon. Mix well and let it simmer for 5 minutes.

4. Put the chicken back into the pan and cover it with the creamy sauce.

5. Serve the chicken drizzled with the sauce on a plate.

STORAGE: Store in an airtight container in the fridge for up to 4 days or in the freezer for up to 1 month.

REHEAT: Microwave, covered, until the desired temperature is reached or reheat in a frying pan or air fryer / instant pot, covered, on medium.

SERVE IT WITH: To make this a complete meal, serve it with a bowl of green salad.

PER SERVING

calories: 395 | fat: 18.2g | total carbs: 1.2g | fiber: 0.3g | protein: 53.7g

Cheesy Low-Carb Chicken

Macros: Fat: 41% | Protein: 54% | Carbs: 5%

Prep time: 10 minutes | Cook time: 1 hour | Serves 4

This cheesy chicken dish is seasoned with oregano and topped with cheese to make a delicious low-carb meal that is perfect for the healthy eaters and kids. It is a family-friendly meal that is perfect for any night of the week.

1 (2- to 3-pound / 0.9- to 1.4-kg) whole chicken, cut into uniform pieces

⅛ cup extra virgin olive oil

1 cup chicken stock

1 clove garlic, crushed

1 teaspoon dried oregano

Salt and freshly ground black pepper, to taste

¼ cup grated Romano cheese

3 tablespoons balsamic vinegar

1. Start by preheating the oven to 450°F (235°C).
2. Put the chicken in a baking dish, then pour the olive oil and chicken stock over it. Sprinkle with the garlic. Season with oregano, salt, and pepper, then scatter the cheese over the chicken.

3. Put the baking dish in the preheated oven to bake for 45 to 60 minutes until cooked through.

4. Remove from the oven and serve the chicken drizzled with the vinegar on a plate.

STORAGE: Store in an airtight container in the fridge for up to 4 days or in the freezer for up to 1 month.

REHEAT: Microwave, covered, until the desired temperature is reached or reheat in a frying pan or air fryer / instant pot, covered, on medium.

SERVE IT WITH: To make this a complete meal, serve it with a bowl of green salad.

PER SERVING

calories: 389 | fat: 17.7g | total carbs: 5.1g | fiber: 0.1g | protein: 52.3g

Sour And Spicy Chicken Breast

Macros: Fat: 45% | Protein: 54% | Carbs: 1%

Prep time: 10 minutes | Cook time: 10 minutes | Serves 4

This delicious chicken breast brings the perfect tangy and spicy combination to any chicken dish. Marinated and grilled, it is perfectly crispy on the outside and juicy on the inside, making it a lip-smacking experience for every tongue.

4 skinless, boneless chicken breast halves

⅛ cup extra virgin olive oil

1 lemon, juiced

2 teaspoons crushed garlic

1 teaspoon salt

1½ teaspoons black pepper

⅓ teaspoon paprika

2 tablespoons olive oil, divided

1. Combine the olive oil, lemon, garlic, salt, pepper, and paprika in a bowl, then set aside.
2. Cut 3 slits into the chicken breasts to allow the marinade to soak in. Put the chicken in a separate bowl and pour the marinade over it.
3. Cover the bowl with plastic wrap and put in the refrigerator to marinate overnight.

4. Preheat the grill to medium heat and brush the grill grates with 1 tablespoon of olive oil.

5. Remove the chicken from the marinade and place it on the grill to cook for about 5 minutes until the juices are clear. Flip the chicken over and brush with the remaining olive oil. Grill for 3 minutes more.

6. Remove the chicken from the grill and serve on plates.

STORAGE: Store in an airtight container in the fridge for up to 4 days or in the freezer for up to 1 month.

REHEAT: Microwave, covered, until the desired temperature is reached or reheat in a frying pan or air fryer / instant pot, covered, on medium.

SERVE IT WITH: To make this a complete meal, serve it with cheesy baked asparagus or creamy cucumber salad.

PER SERVING

calories: 399 | fat: 19.8g | total carbs: 2.1g | fiber: 0.4g | protein: 53.4g

9 781803 176635